Calisthenics Exercises for Beginners

Understanding the Benefits of Calisthenics Exercises

By

Durward Cormac

Copyright@2023

Table of Contents

CHAPTER 1
Introduction

1.1 What Are Calisthenics Exercises?

Calisthenics, often referred to as bodyweight training, is a form of physical exercise that relies primarily on using your own body weight for resistance. It's a fitness discipline that has been practiced for centuries and is rooted in ancient Greece, where it was an integral part of physical education. The term "calisthenics" is derived from the Greek words "kalos," meaning beauty, and "sthenos," meaning strength. Essentially, calisthenics is about developing strength, flexibility, and endurance while emphasizing the harmony of movement and the aesthetics of the human body.

Calisthenics exercises encompass a wide range of movements and techniques that engage various muscle groups. These exercises can be performed almost anywhere, making them incredibly accessible to individuals of all fitness levels. From simple movements like push-ups and squats to more advanced maneuvers like muscle-ups and human flags, calisthenics offers a versatile and effective approach to fitness that doesn't require expensive equipment or gym memberships.

What sets calisthenics apart from traditional weightlifting is its emphasis on functional strength and full-body integration. Calisthenics exercises often mimic natural movements and promote overall athleticism, making it a fantastic choice for beginners who want to build a strong foundation in physical fitness.

1.2 Benefits of Calisthenics for Beginners

Calisthenics is an excellent choice for beginners for several compelling reasons:

1. Accessibility: One of the most significant advantages of calisthenics is its accessibility. You don't need access to a gym or specialized equipment to get started. All you need is your own body and a safe space to train, making it a cost-effective and convenient option for beginners.

2. Full-Body Workout: Calisthenics engages multiple muscle groups simultaneously, providing a full-body workout. This is ideal for beginners who want to develop balanced strength and functional fitness. It helps improve core strength, flexibility, and coordination, which are essential components of overall health.

3. Progressive Overload: Calisthenics allows for a gradual progression of exercises, making it suitable for beginners. You can start with easier variations of movements and gradually advance to more challenging ones as your strength and skill improve. This built-in progression keeps workouts engaging and helps prevent plateaus.

4. Improved Body Composition: For beginners looking to improve their body composition, calisthenics can be highly effective. It helps burn calories, build lean muscle, and increase metabolism, all of which contribute to a healthier body composition.

5. Minimal Risk of Injury: When performed with proper form and technique, calisthenics exercises have a relatively low risk of injury, especially compared to some high-impact sports or weightlifting. This is reassuring for beginners who may be concerned about safety.

6. Enhanced Functional Fitness: Calisthenics doesn't just build muscle; it also improves functional fitness. Everyday activities become easier as your body becomes more agile and adaptable. This can lead to a better quality of life outside the gym.

7. Versatility and Creativity:
Calisthenics allows for endless
variations and creativity in designing
workouts. This versatility keeps
training sessions interesting and can
help beginners stay motivated over
the long term.

8. Mental Benefits: Engaging in
calisthenics can have positive effects
on mental well-being. Exercise
releases endorphins, reducing stress
and boosting mood. Additionally, the
sense of accomplishment that comes
with mastering new calisthenics skills
can boost confidence and self-esteem.

calisthenics is an inclusive and
effective fitness approach that offers
numerous benefits for beginners.
Whether you're aiming to improve
your overall fitness, build muscle, or
simply lead a healthier lifestyle,
calisthenics provides a welcoming

entry point to the world of physical fitness and has the potential to be a lifelong pursuit. This guide will explore calisthenics in depth, providing you with the knowledge and tools to embark on your journey toward a stronger, healthier you.

CHAPTER 2

Getting Started with Calisthenics

2.1 Assessing Your Current Fitness Level

Before diving headfirst into a calisthenics routine, it's essential to assess your current fitness level. This step serves as a crucial baseline, helping you tailor your workouts to your capabilities while preventing overexertion and injury. Here are some key aspects to consider when assessing your fitness level:

- **Strength**: Determine your strength in various muscle groups. How many push-ups, squats, or pull-ups can you do with good form? This will help you identify your starting point.

- **Flexibility**: Assess your flexibility by performing basic stretches. Note any tightness or limitations in your range of motion.

- **Endurance**: Evaluate your cardiovascular endurance by measuring how long you can maintain moderate-intensity activities like jogging, jumping jacks, or planks.

- **Mobility**: Check your joint mobility and range of motion. Are there any areas of stiffness or discomfort?

- **Injuries or Health Concerns**: Consider any past injuries, health conditions, or physical limitations. Consult with a healthcare professional if needed to ensure your safety.

honestly assessing your current fitness level, you can establish a starting point and track your progress effectively. It's important to remember that everyone starts somewhere, and the goal is gradual improvement over time.

2.2 Setting Realistic Goals

Setting clear and realistic goals is a crucial step in your calisthenics journey. Realistic goals help you stay motivated, track your progress, and ensure that your efforts are focused and purposeful. When setting your goals, consider the following tips:

- **Specificity**: Define your goals with precision. Instead of saying, "I want to get fit," specify, "I want to be able to do 10 consecutive push-ups with proper form."

- **Measurable**: Make your goals quantifiable. This allows you to track your progress. For instance, "I want to reduce my 5K run time by 2 minutes."

- **Achievable**: Ensure your goals are attainable based on your current fitness level. Setting overly ambitious goals can lead to frustration and burnout.

- **Relevant**: Your goals should align with your overall fitness aspirations. They should matter to you and contribute to your well-being.

- **Time-Bound**: Set a timeframe for achieving your goals. For example, "I want to achieve 10 pull-ups within six months."

Some examples of realistic calisthenics goals for beginners might include mastering basic exercises like push-ups and squats, increasing endurance in planks, or improving flexibility in specific muscle groups.

2.3 Safety Considerations

Safety should always be a top priority in calisthenics and any fitness endeavor. Here are some safety considerations for beginners:

- **Proper Form**: Learn and practice proper form for each exercise. Incorrect form can lead to injuries and hinder progress.

- **Warm-Up and Cool-Down**: Always warm up before your workouts to prepare your muscles and joints. Similarly, cool down after each session to aid recovery.

- **Gradual Progression**: Avoid rushing into advanced exercises. Gradually progress to more challenging movements to allow your body to adapt.

- **Rest and Recovery**: Give your body adequate time to recover between workouts. Overtraining can lead to injuries and fatigue.

- **Listen to Your Body**: Pay attention to any pain, discomfort, or unusual

sensations during exercises. If
something doesn't feel right,
stop immediately and seek
guidance if necessary.

- **Hydration and Nutrition**:
  Stay hydrated before, during,
  and after your workouts.
  Maintain a balanced diet to
  support your fitness goals.

- **Consult a Professional**: If you
  have any underlying health
  concerns, injuries, or
  uncertainties, consult with a
  fitness professional or
  healthcare provider before
  starting a calisthenics program.

Assessing your fitness level, setting
realistic goals, and prioritizing safety,
you'll lay a solid foundation for your
calisthenics journey. Remember that
progress may be gradual, but each

step forward brings you closer to your fitness objectives.

CHAPTER 3

Warm-Up and Cool-Down

3.1 Importance of Warm-Up

A proper warm-up is essential before engaging in any calisthenics workout. It serves several crucial purposes:

1. **Increased Blood Flow**: A warm-up gradually raises your heart rate, increasing blood flow to your muscles. This helps prepare your body for more intense physical activity.

2. **Muscle Temperature**: Warming up raises the temperature of your muscles,

making them more pliable and less prone to injury. Warm muscles are more efficient and less likely to tear or strain.

3. **Improved Range of Motion**: A warm-up includes dynamic stretches that promote flexibility and joint mobility. This improved range of motion allows you to perform exercises with better form and reduced risk of injury.

4. **Mental Preparation**: A warm-up provides an opportunity to mentally prepare for your workout. It helps you focus, set goals, and establish a positive mindset.

5. **Injury Prevention**: By gradually increasing the intensity of your activity, you

reduce the risk of sudden stress on your muscles, tendons, and ligaments, which can lead to injuries.

3.2 Effective Warm-Up Exercises

An effective warm-up for calisthenics should consist of dynamic exercises that engage various muscle groups and gradually increase in intensity. Here are some warm-up exercises to consider:

1. **Jumping Jacks**: Start with a few minutes of jumping jacks to get your heart rate up and your blood flowing.

2. **Arm Circles**: Stand with your feet hip-width apart and extend your arms straight out. Make

small circular motions with your arms, gradually increasing the size of the circles. Reverse the direction after 1 minute.

3. **Leg Swings**: Stand next to a wall or support, and swing one leg forward and backward, then side to side. This warms up your hip flexors, hamstrings, and quadriceps.

4. **Hip Circles**: Stand with your hands on your hips and make circular motions with your hips, gradually increasing the size of the circles. Change direction after 30 seconds.

5. **Bodyweight Squats**: Perform slow and controlled bodyweight squats to warm up your leg muscles. Focus on proper form.

6. **Arm Swings**: Stand with your feet shoulder-width apart and extend your arms out to the sides. Swing your arms in front of you and then behind you in a controlled manner.

7. **High Knees**: March in place while lifting your knees as high as possible with each step. This engages your hip flexors and warms up your lower body.

8. **Push-Up to Downward Dog**: Perform a push-up and then push back into a downward dog position, stretching your hamstrings and calves.

9. **Plank**: Finish your warm-up with a brief plank hold to engage your core muscles.

3.3 Cooling Down After Your Workout

Cooling down is equally important as warming up. It helps your body transition from intense activity back to a resting state and promotes recovery. Here's why cooling down is crucial:

1. **Reduced Heart Rate**: A cool-down gradually lowers your heart rate, preventing blood pooling in your extremities and helping to stabilize your circulation.

2. **Muscle Recovery**: Stretching during the cool-down can reduce muscle tension and soreness. It aids in the removal of waste products like lactic acid that accumulate during exercise.

3. **Improved Flexibility**:
   Stretching during the cool-
   down helps maintain or
   improve your flexibility, which
   can reduce the risk of injury.

4. **Mental Relaxation**: The cool-
   down is an opportunity to
   mentally unwind and reflect on
   your workout. It can help
   reduce stress and promote a
   sense of well-being.

Effective cooling down after a calisthenics workout includes:

- **Static Stretching**: Hold each stretch for 15-30 seconds. Focus on major muscle groups such as the hamstrings, quadriceps, calves, chest, and shoulders.

- **Deep Breathing**: Spend a few minutes practicing deep,

diaphragmatic breathing to relax your body and reduce post-workout tension.

- **Rehydration**: Rehydrate by drinking water or an electrolyte-rich beverage to replace fluids lost during exercise.

- **Self-Massage**: Consider using a foam roller or a massage stick to release muscle tension.

Cooling down should be a gradual process, lasting about 5-10 minutes, and it should be tailored to your workout intensity. It helps your body recover more effectively, reduces the risk of muscle soreness, and prepares you for your next training session.

CHAPTER 4

Basic Calisthenics Exercises

4.1 Push-Ups

Push-ups are a fundamental calisthenics exercise that targets multiple muscle groups in your upper body, primarily the chest, shoulders, and triceps. Here's how to perform a proper push-up:

1. **Starting Position**: Begin in a plank position with your hands placed slightly wider than shoulder-width apart. Your body should form a straight line from head to heels, and your feet should be hip-width apart.

2. **Execution**: Lower your body by bending your elbows while keeping them close to your torso. Lower yourself until your chest is just above the ground, or as far as your strength allows without compromising form.

3. **Push-Up**: Push your body back up to the starting position by straightening your arms. Keep your core engaged and maintain a straight line from head to heels throughout the movement.

4. **Repetitions**: Perform the desired number of repetitions, focusing on controlled movements and proper form.

Tips:

- Keep your core tight throughout the exercise to maintain a straight body line.

- Ensure your elbows are at a 45-degree angle to your torso as you lower yourself.

- If you're a beginner, you can start with knee push-ups or elevated push-ups (elevating your hands on an elevated surface, like a bench).

4.2 Bodyweight Squats

Bodyweight squats are an excellent lower body exercise that targets the quadriceps, hamstrings, glutes, and calves. Here's how to perform a proper bodyweight squat:

1. **Starting Position**: Stand with your feet shoulder-width apart,

toes pointing slightly outward. Keep your chest up, shoulders back, and your arms extended straight in front of you for balance.

2. **Execution**: Initiate the squat by pushing your hips back and bending your knees. Imagine sitting back into an invisible chair. Keep your weight on your heels as you lower your body.

3. **Squat Down**: Lower your body until your thighs are parallel to the ground or as far as your mobility and strength allow. Ensure your knees are in line with your toes, and your back remains straight.

4. **Squat Up**: Push through your heels to stand back up,

straightening your legs and returning to the starting position.

5. **Repetitions**: Perform the desired number of repetitions, maintaining proper form throughout.

Tips:

- Keep your chest up and your gaze forward during the squat.

- Ensure your knees track in line with your toes and don't collapse inward.

- Control the movement both on the way down and on the way up to work the muscles effectively.

- If you're a beginner, start with partial squats or use a support (like a chair) for balance until you build strength and mobility.

These basic calisthenics exercises, push-ups and bodyweight squats, are foundational movements that can be incorporated into your workouts to build strength and improve overall fitness. As you progress, you can increase the intensity and complexity of these exercises to continue challenging your body and achieving your fitness goals.

4.3 Planks

Planks are a core-strengthening exercise that also engages various muscle groups throughout the body, including the shoulders, back, and legs. Here's how to perform a proper plank:

1. **Starting Position**: Begin in a
   push-up position with your
   hands directly beneath your
   shoulders. Your body should
   form a straight line from head
   to heels, and your feet should
   be hip-width apart.

2. **Execution**: Lower yourself
   onto your forearms, keeping
   your elbows directly beneath
   your shoulders. Your forearms
   should be parallel to each other,
   and your fists or palms should
   be flat on the ground.

3. **Hold the Plank**: Engage your
   core muscles and glutes to lift
   your body off the ground.
   Maintain a straight line from
   head to heels, ensuring your
   hips don't sag or rise too high.
   Keep your neck in line with

your spine, and look at the
ground.

4. **Breathing**: Breathe steadily
   and hold the plank position for
   as long as you can with proper
   form. Aim to start with 20-30
   seconds and gradually increase
   your hold time as you become
   stronger.

5. **Release**: Lower your body back
   to the ground when you can no
   longer maintain proper form.

Tips:

- Focus on engaging your core
  muscles throughout the
  exercise.

- Keep your glutes tight to
  prevent your hips from sagging.

- Avoid holding your breath;
  maintain steady breathing.

- Modify the plank by starting with knee planks if needed.

4.4 Lunges

Lunges are an effective lower body exercise that targets the quadriceps, hamstrings, glutes, and calves. Here's how to perform a basic forward lunge:

1. **Starting Position**: Stand with your feet hip-width apart, and your hands on your hips or by your sides for balance.

2. **Execution**: Take a step forward with one foot, lowering your body by bending both knees. Ensure your front knee is directly above your ankle, and your back knee hovers just above the ground. Your back

heel will be lifted off the ground.

3. **Lunge Down**: Lower your body until your thigh is parallel to the ground or as far as your mobility and strength allow. Keep your upper body upright, and your core engaged.

4. **Step Back**: Push off your front foot and step it back to the starting position. Your feet should return to hip-width apart.

5. **Switch Sides**: Repeat the movement with the other leg to complete one repetition.

6. **Repetitions**: Perform the desired number of repetitions on each leg.

Tips:

- Keep your chest up and your gaze forward during the lunge.

- Ensure your front knee is in line with your toes and doesn't extend beyond them.

- Control the movement on the way down and up to work the muscles effectively.

- Modify the lunge by starting with shorter steps or doing static lunges if you're a beginner.

Planks and lunges are versatile calisthenics exercises that can be incorporated into your fitness routine to strengthen your core, improve balance, and enhance lower body strength. As with any exercise, it's essential to use proper form and gradually increase intensity to avoid injury and maximize results.

4.5 Leg Raises

Leg raises are an excellent calisthenics exercise that primarily targets the abdominal muscles, particularly the lower abs. Here's how to perform leg raises properly:

1. **Starting Position**: Lie on your back on a flat surface, such as a mat, with your legs fully extended and your arms at your sides. Keep your palms facing down, and engage your core muscles.

2. **Execution**: Lift your legs off the ground by flexing your hips and bending your knees slightly. Keep your feet together.

3. **Leg Raise**: Continue raising your legs until they are perpendicular to the ground or

as high as your flexibility allows. Focus on using your lower abdominal muscles to lift your legs.

4. **Lower Legs**: Slowly lower your legs back to the starting position, keeping them controlled and not allowing them to drop suddenly.

5. **Repetitions**: Perform the desired number of repetitions, aiming for controlled movements throughout.

Tips:

- Keep your lower back pressed against the ground to avoid arching it.

- Breathe out as you lift your legs and inhale as you lower them.

- If this exercise is too challenging initially, you can bend your knees more or do knee raises instead.

4.6 Dips

Dips are a compound calisthenics exercise that targets the triceps, shoulders, and chest while also engaging the core and the muscles of the upper back. You can perform dips using parallel bars or a sturdy surface like parallel dip bars or the edge of a stable bench or chair.

Here's how to do parallel bar dips:

1. **Starting Position**: Stand between parallel bars and grab each bar with a firm grip, palms facing down. Keep your arms

fully extended, and your feet together.

2. **Execution**: Lower your body by bending your elbows and leaning forward slightly. Keep your chest up and your shoulders down as you descend.

3. **Dip Down**: Continue descending until your shoulders are slightly below your elbows or as far as your shoulder flexibility allows without discomfort.

4. **Push-Up**: Push your body back up by straightening your arms while exhaling. Focus on using your triceps and chest muscles to lift your body.

5. **Repetitions**: Perform the desired number of repetitions, maintaining proper form.

Tips:

- Keep your body upright, and avoid leaning too far forward or backward.

- Keep your elbows close to your body to emphasize the triceps.

- To make dips easier, you can use an assisted dip machine or place your feet on the ground with your knees bent.

Leg raises and dips are valuable additions to your calisthenics routine. Leg raises target your core muscles, helping you build a strong and toned midsection, while dips work your upper body, particularly the triceps and chest. As with all exercises, focus on using proper form to maximize effectiveness and minimize the risk of injury.

4.7 Wall Sits

Wall sits are a simple yet effective isometric calisthenics exercise that primarily targets the muscles in your lower body, including the quadriceps, hamstrings, glutes, and calf muscles. Wall sits also engage your core for stability. Here's how to perform a wall sit correctly:

1. **Starting Position**: Find a clear wall and stand with your back against it. Your feet should be hip-width apart, and your heels about 1-2 feet away from the wall. Keep your feet flat on the ground.

2. **Execution**: Slowly slide your back down the wall while simultaneously bending your knees. Lower your body until your knees are bent at a 90-degree angle, as if you're sitting in an imaginary chair.

3. **Wall Sit**: Hold this position, ensuring your back remains against the wall, and your thighs are parallel to the ground. Your knees should be directly above your ankles, forming a right angle.

4. **Maintain the Hold**: Engage your core muscles and maintain this seated position for the desired amount of time. Beginners might start with 20-30 seconds and gradually work up to longer holds.

5. **Stand Up**: When you're ready
   to finish, push through your
   heels to stand back up,
   straightening your legs.

Tips:

- Focus on keeping your back
  firmly against the wall
  throughout the exercise.

- Ensure your knees are directly
  above your ankles, and they
  don't extend beyond your toes.

- Breathe steadily and avoid
  holding your breath while
  performing wall sits.

- Increase the difficulty by
  holding weights or a resistance
  band across your thighs.

Wall sits are a fantastic exercise to
build lower body strength, endurance,
and mental toughness. They are often

used in training programs to improve leg stability and arc suitable for people of various fitness levels, making them a valuable addition to your calisthenics routine.

CHAPTER 5

Sample Calisthenics Workouts

5.1 Beginner's Full-Body Workout Routine

This beginner's full-body calisthenics workout is designed to introduce you to fundamental exercises while targeting all major muscle groups. Perform this routine two to three times a week, with at least one rest day in between sessions. As you progress, gradually increase the number of repetitions or duration for each exercise.

Warm-Up (5-10 minutes)

1. **Jumping Jacks**: 2 minutes

   - Stand with feet together and arms at your sides.

   - Jump your feet apart while raising your arms overhead.

   - Return to the starting position and repeat.

2. **Arm Circles**: 2 minutes

   - Stand with feet hip-width apart, extend your arms straight out.

   - Make small circular motions with your arms, gradually increasing the size of the circles.

   - Reverse direction after 1 minute.

3. **Hip Circles**: 1 minute

- Place your hands on your hips and make circular motions with your hips.

- Change direction after 30 seconds.

4. **Bodyweight Squats**: 1 minute

- Perform slow and controlled bodyweight squats to warm up your leg muscles.

Workout Routine

1. **Push-Ups**: 3 sets of 8-10 repetitions

- Start with knee push-ups if needed, and gradually progress to standard push-ups.

2. **Bodyweight Squats**: 3 sets of 12-15 repetitions

- Focus on proper form
  and control throughout
  each squat.

3. **Planks**: 3 sets of 20-30 seconds
hold

- Begin with 20 seconds
  and work your way up to
  longer holds.

4. **Leg Raises**: 3 sets of 8-10
repetitions

- Perform this exercise on
  a mat or the floor with
  proper form.

5. **Wall Sits**: 3 sets of 20-30
seconds hold

- Use proper form and
  engage your core during
  each wall sit.

Cool-Down (5-10 minutes)

1. **Static Stretching**: Hold each stretch for 15-30 seconds.

- Hamstring stretch: Sit on the ground, extend one leg straight, and bend the other leg so the sole of your foot touches your inner thigh. Reach forward to touch your toes.

- Quadriceps stretch: Stand and pull one foot towards your glutes, keeping your knees close together.

- Calf stretch: Step one foot back and press the heel into the ground while keeping the back leg straight.

- Shoulder stretch: Cross one arm over your chest

and gently pull it closer
using your opposite
hand.

- Triceps stretch: Reach
  one arm overhead,
  bending your elbow, and
  use the opposite hand to
  gently push your bent
  elbow.

2. **Deep Breathing**: Spend a few minutes practicing deep, diaphragmatic breathing to relax your body and reduce post-workout tension.

Remember to stay hydrated throughout your workout, and if at any point you experience pain beyond the typical muscle fatigue, stop the exercise and consult a fitness professional or healthcare provider. As you progress, consider adding variations and increasing the intensity of these exercises to continue challenging your body and achieving your fitness goals.

5.2 Upper Body Emphasis Routine

This upper body emphasis calisthenics workout is designed to target and strengthen the muscles of your upper body, including your chest, shoulders, back, and arms. Perform this routine two to three times a week, with at least one rest day in between sessions.

Warm-Up (5-10 minutes)

1. **Jumping Jacks**: 2 minutes

    - Stand with feet together and arms at your sides.

- Jump your feet apart while raising your arms overhead.

- Return to the starting position and repeat.

2. **Arm Circles**: 2 minutes

    - Stand with feet hip-width apart, extend your arms straight out.

    - Make small circular motions with your arms, gradually increasing the size of the circles.

    - Reverse direction after 1 minute.

Workout Routine

1. **Push-Ups**: 4 sets of 8-10 repetitions

- Focus on proper form and control. You can adjust the difficulty by changing hand placement or elevating your feet.

2. **Dips**: 3 sets of 8-10 repetitions

   - Use parallel bars, a sturdy surface, or a dip station for this exercise. Focus on controlled movements.

3. **Pull-Ups or Inverted Rows**: 4 sets of 6-8 repetitions

   - If you have access to a pull-up bar, perform pull-ups. If not, use a sturdy horizontal bar or a suspension trainer for inverted rows.

4. **Push-Up Variations**: 3 sets of 6-8 repetitions each (choose one)

- Diamond push-ups: Place your hands close together to target your triceps.

- Wide push-ups: Widen your hand placement to engage your chest more.

- Archer push-ups: Perform push-ups while shifting your weight from one side to the other to emphasize one arm at a time.

Cool-Down (5-10 minutes)

1. **Static Stretching**: Hold each stretch for 15-30 seconds.

- Chest stretch: Stand with your feet shoulder-width

apart, clasp your hands
behind your back, and
gently lift your arms.

- Shoulder stretch: Extend
  one arm across your
  chest and use your
  opposite hand to gently
  pull it closer.

- Triceps stretch: Reach
  one arm overhead,
  bending your elbow, and
  use the opposite hand to
  gently push your bent
  elbow.

- Neck and upper back
  stretch: Tilt your head to
  one side, holding it with
  your hand for a gentle
  stretch.

2. **Deep Breathing**: Spend a few
   minutes practicing deep,

diaphragmatic breathing to relax your upper body and reduce post-workout tension.

This upper body emphasis routine will help you build strength and endurance in your chest, shoulders, arms, and upper back. As you progress, consider increasing the repetitions or difficulty of exercises to continue challenging yourself and achieving your upper body fitness goals.

5.3 Lower Body Emphasis Routine

This lower body emphasis calisthenics workout is designed to target and strengthen the muscles of your lower body, including your quadriceps, hamstrings, glutes, and calves. Perform this routine two to three times a week, with at least one rest day in between sessions.

Warm-Up (5-10 minutes)

1. **Jumping Jacks**: 2 minutes

    - Stand with feet together and arms at your sides.

    - Jump your feet apart while raising your arms overhead.

    - Return to the starting position and repeat.

2. **Arm Circles**: 2 minutes

    - Stand with feet hip-width apart, extend your arms straight out.

    - Make small circular motions with your arms, gradually increasing the size of the circles.

- Reverse direction after 1 minute.

Workout Routine

1. **Bodyweight Squats**: 4 sets of 12-15 repetitions

   - Focus on proper form and control throughout each squat.

2. **Lunges**: 3 sets of 10-12 repetitions per leg

   - Perform forward or reverse lunges, alternating legs with each repetition.

3. **Wall Sits**: 3 sets of 20-30 seconds hold

   - Engage your core and maintain proper form during each wall sit.

4. **Calf Raises**: 4 sets of 12-15 repetitions

    - Stand with feet hip-width apart, raise onto your toes, and lower back down in a controlled manner.

Cool-Down (5-10 minutes)

1. **Static Stretching**: Hold each stretch for 15-30 seconds.

    - Hamstring stretch: Sit on the ground, extend one leg straight, and bend the other leg so the sole of your foot touches your inner thigh. Reach forward to touch your toes.

    - Quadriceps stretch: Stand and pull one foot towards

your glutes, keeping your knees close together.

- Calf stretch: Step one foot back and press the heel into the ground while keeping the back leg straight.

- Hip flexor stretch: Kneel on one knee, with the other foot in front, and gently press your hips forward.

2. **Deep Breathing**: Spend a few minutes practicing deep, diaphragmatic breathing to relax your lower body and reduce post-workout tension.

This lower body emphasis routine will help you build strength, endurance, and stability in your lower body muscles. As you progress, consider increasing the repetitions or difficulty of exercises to continue challenging yourself and achieving your lower body fitness goals.

CHAPTER 6

Progression and Variations

6.1 How to Progress in Calisthenics

Progression in calisthenics is the key to continuous improvement in strength, endurance, and skill. As you become more proficient in basic exercises, it's important to challenge yourself by increasing the difficulty or intensity of your workouts. Here are some strategies for progressing in calisthenics:

1. **Increase Repetitions**: The simplest way to progress is to perform more repetitions of an

exercise. Gradually increase the number of reps you do for each set until you reach your desired goal.

2. **Modify Exercises**: Modify basic exercises to make them more challenging. For example, you can do push-ups with your feet elevated, perform one-arm push-ups, or try different types of pull-ups (e.g., wide grip, close grip).

3. **Slow Eccentrics**: Focus on the eccentric (lowering) phase of an exercise. For example, during a pull-up, take your time lowering yourself down instead of quickly dropping. This increases time under tension and builds strength.

4. **Isometric Holds**: Incorporate
   isometric holds into your
   routine. For example, in a push-
   up, pause at the bottom position
   before pushing back up.
   Isometric holds build strength
   at specific points in the
   exercise.

5. **Add Weight**: Once you've
   mastered bodyweight exercises,
   consider adding weight to your
   routine. You can use a weight
   vest, dip belt, or hold
   dumbbells or a backpack with
   added weight during exercises
   like squats, dips, or lunges.

6. **Increase Range of Motion**:
   Work on increasing the range
   of motion in your exercises. For
   instance, in a bodyweight squat,
   try to go deeper until your

thighs are parallel to the
ground.

7. **Complex Movements**:
   Combine multiple exercises
   into complex movements. For
   example, you can transition
   from a push-up into a plank,
   then into a side plank for a
   more challenging sequence.

8. **Reduce Rest Time**: Decrease
   the rest time between sets and
   exercises to improve your
   cardiovascular fitness and
   endurance.

9. **Plyometrics**: Integrate
   plyometric exercises like jump
   squats, burpees, and explosive
   push-ups to improve power and
   explosiveness.

10. **Skill Work**: Progression in
    calisthenics often involves

mastering new skills, such as handstands, muscle-ups, or planches. These skills require dedicated practice and gradual progression in their own right.

11. **Periodization**: Implement periodization, which involves cycling through phases of training with varying intensity and volume. For example, you might have a strength-focused phase, followed by a hypertrophy phase, and then a phase focused on skill development.

12. **Track Your Progress**: Keep a workout journal to track your exercises, sets, reps, and progress over time. This allows you to see how far you've come and identify areas for improvement.

13. **Stay Consistent**: Consistency is crucial in calisthenics. Stick to your workout routine, and don't get discouraged if progress is slow at times. Plateaus are normal, but with patience and persistence, you can overcome them.

Safety and proper form should always be a priority when progressing in calisthenics. Avoid attempting exercises or variations that are beyond your current capabilities, as this can lead to injury. Consult with a fitness professional if you're uncertain about how to progress safely or if you encounter any challenges along the way. Progress should be gradual and sustainable, promoting long-term fitness and skill development.

6.2 Advanced Calisthenics Exercises

Once you've built a strong foundation in calisthenics and mastered basic exercises, you can challenge yourself with advanced calisthenics exercises. These movements require a higher level of strength, balance, and control. Here are some advanced calisthenics exercises to consider incorporating into your routine:

1. **Muscle-Ups**: Muscle-ups are a combination of a pull-up and a dip, requiring explosive upper body strength. To perform a muscle-up, start from a dead hang on a pull-up bar, then pull your chest above the bar and transition into a dip.

2. **Front Lever**: The front lever is a gymnastic move that involves

holding your body horizontally while gripping a bar. It requires exceptional core and upper body strength.

3. **Back Lever**: Similar to the front lever, the back lever involves holding your body horizontally, but with your back facing the ground. It's an advanced gymnastic exercise that requires excellent shoulder and core strength.

4. **Human Flag**: The human flag is an iconic calisthenics move where you hold your body horizontally while gripping a vertical pole. It demands immense core and upper body strength, as well as balance.

5. **Planche**: The planche is a static hold where you balance your

body parallel to the ground with only your hands touching the floor. It's a challenging exercise that requires incredible core and shoulder strength.

6. **Handstand Push-Ups**: Handstand push-ups involve performing push-ups while upside down in a handstand position. They target the shoulders, triceps, and core while improving balance and coordination.

7. **One-Arm Push-Ups**: One-arm push-ups are a progression from standard push-ups. You perform a push-up with one hand while balancing on the other. This exercise greatly increases the demand on your chest, triceps, and core.

8. **Dragon Flags**: Dragon flags involve lying on a bench or a stable surface, holding onto the bench behind your head, and lifting your legs and torso in a straight line. This exercise challenges your core and hip flexors.

9. **Pistol Squats**: Pistol squats are one-legged squats where you balance on one leg while extending the other leg straight out in front of you. They require significant leg strength, balance, and flexibility.

10. **L-sits and V-sits**: These exercises involve holding your legs extended straight out in front of you (L-sit) or in a V-shape (V-sit) while gripping parallel bars or the floor. They target the core and hip flexors.

11. **One-Arm Pull-Ups**: One-arm pull-ups arc an advanced progression of pull-ups where you perform the exercise with one arm while gripping the bar with thc other hand.

12. **Clapping Push-Ups**: Clapping push-ups involve pushing off the ground explosively during a push-up and clapping your hands together before catching yourself. They improve upper body power and explosiveness.

13. **Tuck Planche Push-Ups**: This exercise combines the planche and push-up. You perform a push-up while maintaining a tucked planche position, challenging both strength and balance.

Advanced calisthenics exercises should be approached gradually, and proper form is crucial to prevent injuries. It's recommended to consult with a fitness professional or coach when attempting these advanced movements, as they often require specialized progressions and training techniques. Additionally, continue to prioritize safety, and don't rush your progression into advanced exercises.

6.3 Incorporating Equipment (Pull-Up Bar, Resistance Bands, etc.)

Incorporating equipment into your calisthenics routine can add variety, challenge, and versatility to your workouts. Here's how you can use equipment like a pull-up bar, resistance bands, and other tools to enhance your calisthenics training:

1. Pull-Up Bar:

A pull-up bar is a versatile piece of equipment that allows you to target your back, biceps, and other upper body muscles. Here's how to incorporate it into your calisthenics routine:

- **Pull-Ups**: Perform standard pull-ups, chin-ups (palms facing you), wide-grip pull-ups, or close-grip pull-ups to target different muscle groups.

- **Hanging Leg Raises**: Hang from the bar and lift your legs to work your core muscles.

- **L-Sit Pull-Ups**: Combine pull-ups with an L-sit to target both your upper body and core simultaneously.

- **Muscle-Ups**: Use the pull-up bar to practice and master muscle-ups, which combine pull-ups and dips.

2. Parallel Bars:

Parallel bars are great for working on dips, leg raises, and other advanced exercises. You can also use them for beginner-friendly exercises like bench dips.

- **Dips**: Perform parallel bar dips to target your triceps, chest, and shoulders.

- **L-Sits and V-Sits**: Grip the parallel bars and lift your legs into L-sit or V-sit positions for core strengthening.

3. Resistance Bands:

Resistance bands are excellent for adding resistance to your exercises, making them more challenging and effective. You can use them for both upper and lower body workouts.

- **Assisted Pull-Ups and Dips**: Loop a resistance band around the pull-up or dip bar and place your foot or knee in the band to assist with the movement.

- **Banded Push-Ups**: Place a resistance band around your back and hold the ends in your hands while doing push-ups to increase resistance.

- **Squats and Lunges**: Step on a resistance band and hold the other end at shoulder height to add resistance to squats and lunges.

4. Suspension Trainer (TRX):

A suspension trainer is a versatile tool that allows for a wide range of bodyweight exercises, including rows, push-ups, and more.

- **Rows**: Adjust the straps to the desired length and perform rowing exercises to target your back and biceps.

- **Push-Ups**: Use the suspension trainer to add instability to your push-ups, making them more challenging.

- **Pistol Squat Assistance**: Hold onto the straps while doing pistol squats to assist with balance.

5. Yoga Mat:

A yoga mat can provide a comfortable and non-slip surface for your workouts, especially when doing floor exercises like planks, leg raises, and stretches.

- **Planks and Core Exercises**: Use the mat to cushion your elbows or knees during planks and other core exercises.

- **Stretching**: Use the mat for post-workout stretching routines to improve flexibility and prevent injuries.

6. Parallettes:

Parallettes are small, portable bars that can help you perform a variety of advanced calisthenics exercises with greater range of motion.

- **Handstand Push-Ups**: Use parallettes to elevate your hands during handstand push-ups.

- **L-Sits and Planche Progressions**: Parallettes provide better clearance for these advanced exercises.

7. Ankle Weights:

Ankle weights can add resistance to leg exercises, making them more challenging.

- **Leg Raises and Leg Lifts**: Strap ankle weights to your ankles while doing leg raises or leg lifts for added resistance.

When incorporating equipment into your calisthenics routine, remember to prioritize safety and proper form. Start with equipment that matches your current fitness level, and gradually progress as you become more comfortable and stronger. Consult with a fitness professional or trainer if you're unsure about how to use specific equipment or if you need guidance on creating a tailored workout plan.

CHAPTER 7

Common Mistakes to Avoid

Calisthenics is a highly effective and accessible form of exercise, but like any physical activity, it comes with potential pitfalls. Here are some common mistakes to avoid to ensure a safe and productive calisthenics training experience:

7.1 Overtraining

Overtraining occurs when you push your body beyond its capacity for recovery. This can lead to fatigue, injuries, and a plateau in your progress. To avoid overtraining:

- **Stick to a Structured Routine**: Follow a well-designed workout plan with scheduled rest days. Overtraining often happens when people train intensely every day without adequate recovery.

- **Listen to Your Body**: Pay attention to signs of fatigue, soreness, and reduced performance. If you're constantly feeling exhausted or experiencing persistent pain, it's a sign to scale back your training.

- **Prioritize Quality Over Quantity**: More is not always better. Focus on the quality of your exercises and ensure proper form rather than doing excessive repetitions or sets.

- **Include Active Rest**: On rest days, consider low-intensity activities like walking or yoga to keep your body active without overloading it.

7.2 Poor Form

Performing calisthenics exercises with improper form can lead to injuries and hinder your progress. To maintain good form:

- **Learn Proper Technique**: Take the time to learn the correct form for each exercise. Consult tutorials, videos, or a fitness professional to ensure you're performing movements correctly.

- **Start with the Basics**: Master basic exercises before moving on to more advanced variations. Proper form in foundational movements sets the stage for success in advanced calisthenics.

- **Use Mirrors or Recording**: Use mirrors or record your workouts to self-assess your form. This can help you identify and correct any form flaws.

- **Engage Core and Stabilizers**: Proper form often involves engaging your core and stabilizer muscles to maintain balance and control during exercises.

7.3 Neglecting Rest and Recovery

Rest and recovery are essential components of any training program. Neglecting them can lead to burnout, injuries, and a lack of progress. To prioritize rest and recovery:

- **Schedule Rest Days**: Incorporate scheduled rest days into your training plan. These days allow your muscles and nervous system to recover.

- **Prioritize Sleep**: Ensure you're getting enough quality sleep, as it's crucial for muscle repair and overall recovery.

- **Nutrition**: Fuel your body with a balanced diet to support your training and recovery. Adequate protein intake is especially important for muscle repair.

- **Hydration**: Stay well-hydrated to support your body's recovery processes.

- **Active Recovery**: On rest days, consider light activities like stretching, mobility work, or foam rolling to aid recovery.

- **Listen to Your Body**: If you're feeling fatigued, sore, or unmotivated, it's okay to adjust your training or take an extra rest day. Your body knows when it needs recovery.

- **Avoid Overloading**: Don't pack too many exercises into a single session. Allow enough time between sets and exercises to recover and perform each movement with proper form.

By avoiding these common mistakes, you'll be able to enjoy a safe and effective calisthenics training journey that yields steady progress and keeps you injury-free. Remember that consistency, patience, and a balanced approach to training are key to long-term success in calisthenics.

CHAPTER 8

Nutrition and Diet Tips

8.1 Importance of Nutrition in Calisthenics

Nutrition plays a pivotal role in your calisthenics performance, recovery, and overall fitness journey. Here's why nutrition is crucial for calisthenics:

1. **Energy Source**: Your body needs energy (calories) to fuel workouts and daily activities. Proper nutrition ensures you have the energy required to perform your best during calisthenics sessions.

2. **Muscle Repair and Growth**:
   After intense calisthenics
   exercises, your muscles require
   nutrients, especially protein, to
   repair and grow stronger.
   Adequate protein intake
   supports muscle recovery and
   development.

3. **Recovery**: Nutrition plays a
   vital role in post-workout
   recovery. Consuming the right
   nutrients can reduce muscle
   soreness, promote faster
   recovery, and prepare you for
   the next training session.

4. **Optimal Performance**: Proper
   nutrition provides your body
   with essential vitamins,
   minerals, and micronutrients
   that are crucial for maintaining
   overall health and maximizing
   your calisthenics performance.

5. **Body Composition**: Nutrition plays a significant role in achieving and maintaining a healthy body composition. Balancing calories in versus calories out can help with weight management and body fat reduction.

6. **Hydration**: Staying well-hydrated is essential for optimal muscle function, joint lubrication, and overall performance. Dehydration can lead to decreased exercise capacity and increased risk of injury.

8.2 Pre-Workout and Post-Workout Nutrition

Pre-Workout Nutrition:

Before your calisthenics workout, consider these guidelines for pre-workout nutrition:

- **Carbohydrates**: Consume complex carbohydrates like whole grains, fruits, or vegetables 1-2 hours before exercise. Carbs provide energy for your workout.

- **Protein**: Include a moderate amount of protein to help prevent muscle breakdown during exercise. Options like yogurt, nuts, or a protein shake can be suitable choices.

- **Hydration**: Drink enough water to stay adequately hydrated before your workout.

- **Avoid Heavy Meals**: Avoid large, heavy meals close to your workout to prevent discomfort. Opt for smaller, easily digestible snacks if necessary.

- **Caffeine**: Some people find that a moderate amount of caffeine from sources like coffee or green tea can enhance workout performance and focus.

Post-Workout Nutrition:

After your calisthenics session, focus on post-workout nutrition to aid recovery:

- **Protein**: Consume a protein source (e.g., lean meats, dairy, tofu, legumes, or a protein shake) to promote muscle repair and growth.

- **Carbohydrates**: Replenish glycogen stores with carbohydrates to support energy recovery. A combination of protein and carbs in a post-workout meal or snack can be effective.

- **Hydration**: Rehydrate by drinking water or an electrolyte-rich beverage to replace fluids lost during exercise.

- **Timing**: Aim to eat within 1-2 hours after your workout to maximize recovery benefits.

8.3 Hydration

Hydration is essential for calisthenics and overall well-being. Proper hydration helps you maintain peak performance, avoid muscle cramps, and prevent heat-related illnesses. Here are hydration tips:

- **Water Intake**: Drink water throughout the day to stay well-hydrated. The exact amount varies depending on factors like body size, activity level, and climate, but a general guideline is about 8 cups (64 ounces) for adults.

- **Pre-Workout Hydration**: Start your workout session well-hydrated by drinking water in the hours leading up to exercise.

- **During Exercise**: Depending on the duration and intensity of your calisthenics session, consider sipping water during breaks to stay hydrated. For longer or more intense workouts, an electrolyte sports drink can help replace lost minerals like sodium and potassium.

- **Post-Workout Rehydration**: After exercise, continue to drink water to replace fluids lost through sweat. Pay attention to your body's signals of thirst.

- **Electrolytes**: In very hot or humid conditions, or during longer workouts, you may need to replenish electrolytes. Sports drinks, coconut water, or electrolyte tablets can help maintain electrolyte balance.

- **Urine Color**: Monitor the color of your urine as an indicator of hydration. Pale yellow or light straw-colored urine generally indicates proper hydration, while dark yellow or amber urine may suggest dehydration.

Individual hydration needs vary, so it's important to listen to your body. Staying consistently hydrated is key to supporting your calisthenics performance and overall health.

CHAPTER 9

Tracking Your Progress

9.1 Keeping a Workout Journal

Keeping a workout journal is a valuable tool for tracking your progress in calisthenics. It provides a structured way to record your workouts, measure your performance, and make informed adjustments to your training plan. Here's how to maintain an effective workout journal:

1. **Choose a Journal**: Select a dedicated notebook, digital app, or spreadsheet to serve as your

workout journal. It should be easily accessible and organized.

2. **Record Workouts**: After each workout, jot down the details. Include the date, exercises performed, sets, repetitions, and any additional notes (e.g., how you felt, variations attempted).

3. **Track Progress**: Use your journal to monitor improvements in strength, endurance, and skill level. For example, note when you increase the number of repetitions, add weight, or achieve a new exercise variation.

4. **Document Rest and Recovery**: Record your rest days, as well as any changes in sleep patterns, nutrition, and

recovery techniques. This helps you identify factors influencing your progress.

5. **Include Goals**: Set specific, achievable goals for your calisthenics journey. Regularly review your goals and adjust them as you make progress.

6. **Analyze Patterns**: Periodically review your journal to identify patterns or trends. For instance, you might notice that certain exercises are consistently improving, while others are plateauing.

7. **Learn from Setbacks**: Note setbacks or injuries and document how you addressed them. This information can help you prevent similar issues in the future.

8. **Nutrition and Hydration**: Consider recording basic nutrition information, such as meals consumed before workouts, to assess how diet influences your performance.

9. **Motivation and Insights**: Use your journal to jot down motivational quotes, thoughts, or insights that inspire you to keep pushing forward.

10. **Consistency**: The act of recording your workouts can also serve as a motivator to maintain consistency in your training.

9.2 Measuring Results

Measuring results in calisthenics involves assessing your progress over time to determine whether your training is effective. Here's how to measure results effectively:

1. **Physical Measurements**: Track changes in body measurements, such as waist size, chest circumference, and muscle girth. Progress photos taken from multiple angles can also be valuable for visual assessment.

2. **Strength and Performance**: Regularly assess your strength gains by monitoring the number of repetitions and sets you can complete, the resistance or weight used, and your ability to perform advanced exercises.

3. **Skill Development**: Measure your progress in mastering advanced calisthenics skills.

For example, note the duration of your static holds (e.g., plank, L-sit) or the successful execution of complex movements (e.g., muscle-ups).

4. **Endurance**: Evaluate your endurance by tracking improvements in how long you can maintain certain exercises, such as planks, wall sits, or cardio-intensive calisthenics routines.

5. **Rest and Recovery**: Monitor how quickly you recover from workouts and whether you experience reduced soreness over time. This can indicate improved fitness.

6. **Nutrition and Body Composition**: Consider using body composition

measurements, such as body fat percentage, to assess changes in your physique.

7. **Mental and Emotional Well-Being**: Pay attention to your mental and emotional state. Reduced stress levels, improved focus, and increased confidence can be indicators of progress.

8. **Goal Achievement**: Regularly evaluate your progress toward achieving your calisthenics goals. Celebrate milestones and adjust your goals as needed to maintain motivation.

9. **Workout Journal**: Refer to your workout journal to review past workouts, track progress, and identify areas where you've

made significant gains or encountered challenges.

10. **Feedback and Coaching**: Seek feedback from a coach, trainer, or experienced calisthenics practitioner to gain an objective perspective on your progress and receive guidance on areas for improvement.

Progress in calisthenics can be gradual, and plateaus are common. Consistency, patience, and diligent tracking of your workouts and results are key to achieving your fitness goals and continually advancing in your calisthenics journey.

www.ingramcontent.com/pod-product-compliance
Lightning Source LLC
Chambersburg PA
CBHW070820260726
48660CB00005B/1929